Self-Love Journal

MAVEN PRESS

First published in Australia in 2024
by Maven Press
Roleystone WA 6111

NATIONAL LIBRARY OF AUSTRALIA

A catalogue record for this work is available from the National Library of Australia

National Library of Australia Catalogue-in-Publication

data: Self-Love Journal: Maven Press

ISBN: 978-0-9756174-0-3

(Paperback)

Self-Love

Introduction

This self-love journal is more than a collection of blank pages. It's a sacred space designed to be your companion on the transformative voyage to self-love and acceptance.

Each page invites you to explore the depths of your heart, celebrate your triumphs, and embrace your authentic self.

This journal is a sanctuary where self-reflection meets affirmation, where the whispers of self-love echo through the ink on the pages.

As you embark on this guided journey, may these words and reflections become the mirror that reveals the beauty within, leading you to a profound and unshakable love for the incredible person you are and always have been.

Self-Love

Self-Love

Date:

How do I feel today?

What am I grateful for today?

What are my intentions today?

Self-love activities ...

What I accomplished today

Reflection

Self-Love

Self-Love

Self-Love

Self-Love

Self-Love

Self-Love

Date:

How do I feel today?

What am I grateful for today?

What are my intentions today?

Self-love activities ...

What I accomplished today

Reflection

Self-Love

Self-Love

Self-Love

Self-Love

Self-Love

Self-Love

Date:

How do I feel today?

What am I grateful for today?

What are my intentions today?

Self-love activities ...

What I accomplished today

Reflection

Self-Love

Self-Love

Self-Love

Self-Love

Self-Love

Self-Love

Date:

How do I feel today?

What I accomplished today

What am I grateful for today?

What are my intentions today?

Reflection

Self-love activities ...

Self-Love

Self-Love

Self-Love

Self-Love

Self-Love

Self-Love

Date:

How do I feel today?

What am I grateful for today?

What are my intentions today?

Self-love activities ...

What I accomplished today

Reflection

Self-Love

Self-Love

Self-Love

Self-Love

Self-Love

Self-Love

Date:

How do I feel today?

What am I grateful for today?

What are my intentions today?

Self-love activities ...

What I accomplished today

Reflection

Self-Love

Self-Love

Self-Love

Self-Love

Self-Love

Self-Love

Date:

How do I feel today?

What am I grateful for today?

What are my intentions today?

Self-love activities ...

What I accomplished today

Reflection

Self-Love

Self-Love

Self-Love

Self-Love

Self-Love

Self-Love

Date:

How do I feel today?

What am I grateful for today?

What are my intentions today?

Self-love activities ...

What I accomplished today

Reflection

Self-Love

Self-Love

Self-Love

Self-Love

Self-Love

Self-Love

Date:

How do I feel today?

What am I grateful for today?

What are my intentions today?

Self-love activities ...

What I accomplished today

Reflection

Self-Love

Self-Love

Self-Love

Self-Love

Self-Love

Self-Love

Date:

How do I feel today?

What am I grateful for today?

What are my intentions today?

Self-love activities ...

What I accomplished today

Reflection

Self-Love

Self-Love

Self-Love

Self-Love

Self-Love

Self-Love

Date:

How do I feel today?

What am I grateful for today?

What are my intentions today?

Self-love activities ...

What I accomplished today

Reflection

Self-Love

Self-Love

Self-Love

Self-Love

Self-Love

Self-Love

Date:

How do I feel today?

What am I grateful for today?

What are my intentions today?

Self-love activities ...

What I accomplished today

Reflection

Self-Love

Self-Love

Self-Love

Self-Love

Self-Love

Self-Love

Date:

How do I feel today?

What am I grateful for today?

What are my intentions today?

Self-love activities ...

What I accomplished today

Reflection

Self-Love

Self-Love

Self-Love

Self-Love

Self-Love

Self-Love

Date:

How do I feel today?

What am I grateful for today?

What are my intentions today?

Self-love activities ...

What I accomplished today

Reflection

Self-Love

Self-Love

Self-Love

Self-Love

Self-Love

Self-Love

Date:

How do I feel today?

What am I grateful for today?

What are my intentions today?

Self-love activities ...

What I accomplished today

Reflection

Self-Love

Self-Love

Self-Love

Self-Love

Self-Love

Self-Love

Date:

How do I feel today?

What am I grateful for today?

What are my intentions today?

Self-love activities ...

What I accomplished today

Reflection

Self-Love

Self-Love

Self-Love

Self-Love

Self-Love

Self-Love

Date:

How do I feel today?

What I accomplished today

What am I grateful for today?

What are my intentions today?

Reflection

Self-love activities ...

Self-Love

Self-Love

Self-Love

Self-Love

Self-Love

Self-Love

Date:

How do I feel today?

What am I grateful for today?

What are my intentions today?

Self-love activities ...

What I accomplished today

Reflection

Self-Love

Self-Love

Self-Love

Self-Love

Self-Love

Self-Love

Date:

How do I feel today?

What am I grateful for today?

What are my intentions today?

Self-love activities ...

What I accomplished today

Reflection

Self-Love

Self-Love

Self-Love

Self-Love

Self-Love

Self-Love

Date:

How do I feel today?

What am I grateful for today?

What are my intentions today?

Self-love activities ...

What I accomplished today

Reflection

Self-Love

Self-Love

Self-Love

Self-Love

Self-Love

Self-Love

Date:

How do I feel today?

What am I grateful for today?

What are my intentions today?

Self-love activities …

What I accomplished today

Reflection

Self-Love

Self-Love

Self-Love

Self-Love

Self-Love

Self-Love

Date:

How do I feel today?

What am I grateful for today?

What are my intentions today?

Self-love activities ...

What I accomplished today

Reflection

Self-Love

Self-Love

Self-Love

Self-Love

Self-Love

Self-Love

Date:

How do I feel today?

What am I grateful for today?

What are my intentions today?

Self-love activities ...

What I accomplished today

Reflection

Self-Love

Self-Love

Self-Love

Self-Love

Self-Love

Self-Love

Date:

How do I feel today?

What am I grateful for today?

What are my intentions today?

Self-love activities ...

What I accomplished today

Reflection

Self-Love

Self-Love

Self-Love

Self-Love

Self-Love

Self-Love

Date:

How do I feel today?

What am I grateful for today?

What are my intentions today?

Self-love activities ...

What I accomplished today

Reflection

Self-Love

Self-Love

Self-Love

Self-Love

Self-Love

Self-Love

Date:

How do I feel today?

What am I grateful for today?

What are my intentions today?

Self-love activities ...

What I accomplished today

Reflection

Self-Love

Self-Love

Self-Love

Self-Love

Self-Love

Self-Love

Date:

How do I feel today?

What am I grateful for today?

What are my intentions today?

Self-love activities ...

What I accomplished today

Reflection

Self-Love

Self-Love

Self-Love

Self-Love

Self-Love

Self-Love

Date:

How do I feel today?

What am I grateful for today?

What are my intentions today?

Self-love activities ...

What I accomplished today

Reflection

Self-Love

Self-Love

Self-Love

Self-Love

Self-Love

Self-Love

Date:

How do I feel today?

What am I grateful for today?

What are my intentions today?

Self-love activities ...

What I accomplished today

Reflection

Self-Love

Self-Love

Self-Love

Self-Love

Self-Love

Self-Love

Date:

How do I feel today?

What am I grateful for today?

What are my intentions today?

Self-love activities ...

What I accomplished today

Reflection

Self-Love

Self-Love

Self-Love

Self-Love

Self-Love

Self-Love

Date:

How do I feel today?

What am I grateful for today?

What are my intentions today?

Self-love activities ...

What I accomplished today

Reflection

Self-Love

Self-Love

Self-Love

Self-Love

Self-Love

Self-Love

Date:

How do I feel today?

What am I grateful for today?

What are my intentions today?

Self-love activities ...

What I accomplished today

Reflection

Self-Love

Self-Love

Self-Love

Self-Love

Self-Love

Self-Love

Self-Love

Self-Love

www.ingramcontent.com/pod-product-compliance
Lightning Source LLC
Chambersburg PA
CBHW080359030426
42334CB00024B/2927
9780975617403